The Ultimate Wellness Journal for Women

A HOLISTIC APPROACH TO HEALTH

Rachel Russell

SoulSpark Publication

Disclaimer: This book is not intended to diagnose, treat, or cure any illness, disease, or medical problem. No guarantee is made regarding results achieved. The user should consult a medical professional regarding any symptoms of concern or health related issues.

2nd Edition October 2016
Previously published
under the title "The Ultimate Symptom Journal for Women"
SoulSpark Publication
www.soulsparkpublication.com
All rights reserved.
ISBN: 153943639X
ISBN-13: 978-1539436393

*Dedicated to my husband
and children, who have surrounded me
with love and support.*

*And to my mother
who taught me the value
of asking questions and searching
for answers.*

ACKNOWLEDGEMENT

I want to thank the amazing women who have inspired me and participated with me on this adventure: Amie, Ardie, Cary, Connie, Dana, Jenne, Jessica, Kathy, Kim, Leah, Mindy, Pam, Tara, and Zephyr.

Your body is trying to communicate with you. The symptoms we experience are vital messages that we often do not hear until we see them collectively. Writing them down allows you to do just that. Have you ever sat down with a new patient or patient-update form, reading and re-reading the questions, wondering how to answer them? Have you found yourself tired, anxious, irritable, fatigued or overweight, but do not know how to articulate specifics to your doctor? Are you uncertain or unable to answer your doctor's questions regarding your symptoms? You know that you have something to say in regard to each question, but you just can't quite remember the details. Everything has blended together and having meaningful input or precise answers to your healthcare provider's questions becomes impossible.

This eight-week journal is designed to document and prompt you to record relevant information your healthcare provider needs to give you the most complete care.

Whether you are experiencing perimenopause, thyroid dysfunction, chronic migraines, or other issues, taking the time to keep a written record is imperative. As you begin treatment, it will also help you detect subtle improvements in your symptoms. It will also allow you to document your health status and overall actions on a daily basis.

HOW TO USE THIS JOURNAL: You can start on any day of the week or month; this journal is designed to span a full eight weeks. It can be used to document symptoms prior to treatment, during treatment, and after treatment. Take it with you to your appointments with your healthcare provider. Most of the entry prompts are self-explanatory, but here are a few notes on use:

Body Composition & Measurements: Measure at weeks 1, 4, and 8. It is important to focus on measurements and body fat percentage over just weight. For body fat percentage, there are multiple tools that could be used, with varying degrees of accuracy. Whichever you use, stay consistent and use the same one, at the same time of day. Options include calipers, bioelectrical impedance, and others.

Body temperature: Use a non-mercury, non-digital thermometer, leaving it under your tongue for at least 3 minutes. Between uses, you will need to "shake it down" – it will not zero out on its own, or go down even if placed in cold water. Body temperature provides important information regarding thyroid, adrenal, and metabolic function.

Bowel movements: Record how many and any irregularities/ discomfort in bowel movements. The reality is that our bowel movements can reveal a lot about how our system is functioning.

Circadian Rhythm and Metabolic Clock: This section includes a variety of items to track that relate to circadian rhythm and metabolic function.

Daytime activity: Record what types of everyday movement you have, such as sitting at a desk, cleaning house, running errands, a long car ride, etc. It is for non-exercise activity.

Difficulty falling back to sleep: Note any difficulties: anxiety, worry, alertness, etc.

Evening blue light blocking: If you stop using all electronic/digital screens three hours prior to sleep and/or take steps to block blue light (such as filtering glasses), note that here. Why is that important? Evening blue light exposure disrupts our body's natural sleep cycle.

Menstrual cycle: Day 1 is the first full day of your period.

Mood narrative: Record how you feel in regards to any irritability, anxiety, depression, sadness, etc.

Morning sunlight: Document any minutes of exposure to bright morning light or the use of a full spectrum light. Full spectrum light in the morning signals the brain and subsequently, metabolic processes in the body.

Other notes: Anything else that is pertinent such as supplement or medication changes. Were you sick? Using coffee to stay awake? Having cravings for sweets or carbs? (Be specific- which ones?)

Are you wanting to use alcohol or smoking to cope? Dry skin? Thinning Hair? Rashes? Loss of appetite or increased appetite?

Restoration/Relaxation Activities: Deep breathing, meditation, affirmations, yoga, Epsom salt bath, progressive muscle relaxation, etc. Record what you do and for how long.

Time it took to fall asleep: Did you lie awake for an hour staring at the ceiling? Or did you lay down and promptly relax and fall asleep?

GETTING STARTED: Identify below the key obstacles you are facing and what goal you have in pursuing treatment. For example, have you been working out, eating right, but not losing weight? Have you found yourself moody, snapping at family members? Do you find yourself unable to stay awake in the afternoon or spend all evening craving sweets?

_____

_____

_____

_____

_____

_____

_____

_____

Week 1

Date: _May 21/19_

Body Composition & Measurements:
Chest: _40.5_   Waist: _38 -at bellybutton_

Bicep:_____ Hips: _41_

Thigh: _24_   Calf: _14.5_

Body Fat percentage:_____Weight:_161.4_

Circadian Rhythm & Metabolic Clock:

Hours of sleep:_____Time it took to fall asleep:_____

Number of night wakings:_____

Explain any difficulty falling back asleep:_____

_____

Wake-up time:_____ Sleep quality:_____

_____

Wake up feeling rested: Yes   No

Morning body temperature: _____   Time taken: _____

Morning energy level:_____Morning sunlight:_____

Day of menstrual cycle:_____ Daytime activity:_____

Mid-day body temperature:_____ Time taken:_____

Mood Narrative:_____

_____

_____

_____

Afternoon Energy level:_____Bowel movements:_____

_____

Headache/joint pain/other pain symptoms:_____

_____

6

_____

_____

_____

Exercise activity and duration:_____

Relaxation/restoration activities:_____

_____

Evening blue light blocking: Yes   No

Evening/Bedtime hunger:_____

Evening body temperature:_____   Time taken:_____

Bedtime:_____ Libido:_____

Nutrition:

Breakfast time:_____Food:_____

_____

Snack time:_____Food:_____

Lunch time:_____Food:_____

_____

Snack time:_____Food:_____

Dinner time:_____Food:_____

_____

Snack time:_____Food:_____

Daily water intake total:_____

Other notes:_____

_____

_____

_____

_____

Date:_____

Circadian Rhythm & Metabolic Clock:

Hours of sleep:_____Time it took to fall asleep:_____

Number of night wakings:_____

Explain any difficulty falling back asleep:_____

_____

Wake-up time:_____ Sleep quality:_____

_____

Wake up feeling rested: Yes   No

Morning body temperature: _____   Time taken: _____

Morning energy level:_____Morning sunlight:_____

Day of menstrual cycle:_____ Daytime activity:_____

Mid-day body temperature:_____ Time taken:_____

Mood Narrative:_____

_____

_____

_____

_____

Afternoon Energy level:_____Bowel movements:_____

_____

Headache/joint pain/other pain symptoms:_____

_____

_____

_____

_____

Exercise activity and duration:_____

Relaxation/restoration activities:_____

_____

Evening blue light blocking: Yes   No

Evening/Bedtime hunger:_____

Evening body temperature:_____   Time taken:_____

Bedtime:_____ Libido:_____

Nutrition:

Breakfast time:_____Food:_____

_____

Snack time:_____Food:_____

Lunch time:_____Food:_____

_____

Snack time:_____Food:_____

Dinner time:_____Food:_____

_____

Snack time:_____Food:_____

Daily water intake total:_____

Other notes:_____

_____

_____

_____

_____

_____

_____

_____

Date:_____

Circadian Rhythm & Metabolic Clock:

Hours of sleep:_____Time it took to fall asleep:_____

Number of night wakings:_____

Explain any difficulty falling back asleep:_____

_____

Wake-up time:_____ Sleep quality:_____

_____

Wake up feeling rested: Yes   No

Morning body temperature: _____   Time taken: _____

Morning energy level:_____Morning sunlight:_____

Day of menstrual cycle:_____ Daytime activity:_____

Mid-day body temperature:_____ Time taken:_____

Mood Narrative:_____

_____

_____

_____

_____

Afternoon Energy level:_____Bowel movements:_____

_____

Headache/joint pain/other pain symptoms:_____

_____

_____

_____

_____

Exercise activity and duration:_____

Relaxation/restoration activities:_____

_____

Evening blue light blocking: Yes   No

Evening/Bedtime hunger:_____

Evening body temperature:_____   Time taken:_____

Bedtime:_____ Libido:_____

Nutrition:

Breakfast time:_____Food:_____

_____

Snack time:_____Food:_____

Lunch time:_____Food:_____

_____

Snack time:_____Food:_____

Dinner time:_____Food:_____

_____

Snack time:_____Food:_____

Daily water intake total:_____

Other notes:_____

_____

_____

_____

_____

_____

_____

_____

_____

Date:_____

Circadian Rhythm & Metabolic Clock:

Hours of sleep:_____Time it took to fall asleep:_____

Number of night wakings:_____

Explain any difficulty falling back asleep:_____

_____

Wake-up time:_____ Sleep quality:_____

_____

Wake up feeling rested: Yes   No

Morning body temperature: _____   Time taken: _____

Morning energy level:_____Morning sunlight:_____

Day of menstrual cycle:_____ Daytime activity:_____

Mid-day body temperature:_____ Time taken:_____

Mood Narrative:_____

_____

_____

_____

_____

Afternoon Energy level:_____Bowel movements:_____

_____

Headache/joint pain/other pain symptoms:_____

_____

_____

_____

_____

Exercise activity and duration:_____

Relaxation/restoration activities:_____

_____

Evening blue light blocking: Yes   No

Evening/Bedtime hunger:_____

Evening body temperature:_____   Time taken:_____

Bedtime:_____ Libido:_____

Nutrition:

Breakfast time:_____Food:_____

_____

Snack time:_____Food:_____

Lunch time:_____Food:_____

_____

Snack time:_____Food:_____

Dinner time:_____Food:_____

_____

Snack time:_____Food:_____

Daily water intake total:_____

Other notes:_____

_____

_____

_____

_____

_____

_____

_____

_____

Date:_____

Circadian Rhythm & Metabolic Clock:

Hours of sleep:_____Time it took to fall asleep:_____

Number of night wakings:_____

Explain any difficulty falling back asleep:_____

_____

Wake-up time:_____ Sleep quality:_____

_____

Wake up feeling rested: Yes   No

Morning body temperature: _____   Time taken: _____

Morning energy level:_____Morning sunlight:_____

Day of menstrual cycle:_____ Daytime activity:_____

Mid-day body temperature:_____ Time taken:_____

Mood Narrative:_____

_____

_____

_____

_____

Afternoon Energy level:_____Bowel movements:_____

_____

Headache/joint pain/other pain symptoms:_____

_____

_____

_____

_____

Exercise activity and duration:_____

Relaxation/restoration activities:_____

_____

Evening blue light blocking: Yes   No

Evening/Bedtime hunger:_____

Evening body temperature: _____   Time taken:_____

Bedtime:_____ Libido:_____

Nutrition:

Breakfast time:_____Food:_____

_____

Snack time:_____Food:_____

Lunch time:_____Food:_____

_____

Snack time:_____Food:_____

Dinner time:_____Food:_____

_____

Snack time:_____Food:_____

Daily water intake total:_____

Other notes:_____

_____

_____

_____

_____

_____

_____

_____

_____

Date:_____

Circadian Rhythm & Metabolic Clock:

Hours of sleep:_____Time it took to fall asleep:_____

Number of night wakings:_____

Explain any difficulty falling back asleep:_____

_____

Wake-up time:_____ Sleep quality:_____

_____

Wake up feeling rested: Yes   No

Morning body temperature: _____   Time taken: _____

Morning energy level:_____Morning sunlight:_____

Day of menstrual cycle:_____ Daytime activity:_____

Mid-day body temperature:_____ Time taken:_____

Mood Narrative:_____

_____

_____

_____

_____

Afternoon Energy level:_____Bowel movements:_____

_____

Headache/joint pain/other pain symptoms:_____

_____

_____

_____

_____

Exercise activity and duration:_____

Relaxation/restoration activities:_____

_____

Evening blue light blocking: Yes   No

Evening/Bedtime hunger:_____

Evening body temperature: _____   Time taken:_____

Bedtime:_____ Libido:_____

Nutrition:

Breakfast time:_____Food:_____

_____

Snack time:_____Food:_____

Lunch time:_____Food:_____

_____

Snack time:_____Food:_____

Dinner time:_____Food:_____

_____

Snack time:_____Food:_____

Daily water intake total:_____

Other notes:_____

_____

_____

_____

_____

_____

_____

_____

_____

Date:_____

Circadian Rhythm & Metabolic Clock:

Hours of sleep:_____Time it took to fall asleep:_____

Number of night wakings:_____

Explain any difficulty falling back asleep:_____

_____

Wake-up time:_____ Sleep quality:_____

_____

Wake up feeling rested: Yes   No

Morning body temperature: _____ Time taken: _____

Morning energy level:_____Morning sunlight:_____

Day of menstrual cycle:_____ Daytime activity:_____

Mid-day body temperature:_____ Time taken:_____

Mood Narrative:_____

_____

_____

_____

_____

Afternoon Energy level:_____Bowel movements:_____

_____

Headache/joint pain/other pain symptoms:_____

_____

_____

_____

_____

Exercise activity and duration:_____

Relaxation/restoration activities:_____

_____

Evening blue light blocking: Yes   No

Evening/Bedtime hunger:_____

Evening body temperature: _____   Time taken:_____

Bedtime:_____ Libido:_____

Nutrition:

Breakfast time:_____Food:_____

_____

Snack time:_____Food:_____

Lunch time:_____Food:_____

_____

Snack time:_____Food:_____

Dinner time:_____Food:_____

_____

Snack time:_____Food:_____

Daily water intake total:_____

Other notes:_____

_____

_____

_____

_____

_____

_____

_____

Week 1 Summary

What went well:_____

_____

_____

_____

_____

_____

What didn't go so well:_____

_____

_____

_____

_____

_____

Any patterns or potential cause/effect relationships:_____

_____

_____

_____

_____

Questions to ask my doctor:_____

_____

_____

Week 2

Date:_____

Circadian Rhythm & Metabolic Clock:

Hours of sleep:_____Time it took to fall asleep:_____

Number of night wakings:_____

Explain any difficulty falling back asleep:_____

_____

Wake-up time:_____ Sleep quality:_____

_____

Wake up feeling rested: Yes   No

Morning body temperature: _____   Time taken: _____

Morning energy level:_____Morning sunlight:_____

Day of menstrual cycle:_____ Daytime activity:_____

Mid-day body temperature:_____ Time taken:_____

Mood Narrative:_____

_____

_____

_____

_____

Afternoon Energy level:_____Bowel movements:_____

_____

Headache/joint pain/other pain symptoms:_____

_____

_____

_____

_____

Exercise activity and duration:_____

Relaxation/restoration activities:_____

_____

Evening blue light blocking: Yes   No

Evening/Bedtime hunger:_____

Evening body temperature: _____   Time taken:_____

Bedtime:_____ Libido:_____

Nutrition:

Breakfast time:_____Food:_____

_____

Snack time:_____Food:_____

Lunch time:_____Food:_____

_____

Snack time:_____Food:_____

Dinner time:_____Food:_____

_____

Snack time:_____Food:_____

Daily water intake total:_____

Other notes:_____

_____

_____

_____

_____

_____

_____

_____

Date:_____

Circadian Rhythm & Metabolic Clock:

Hours of sleep:_____Time it took to fall asleep:_____

Number of night wakings:_____

Explain any difficulty falling back asleep:_____

_____

Wake-up time:_____ Sleep quality:_____

_____

Wake up feeling rested: Yes   No

Morning body temperature: _____   Time taken: _____

Morning energy level:_____Morning sunlight:_____

Day of menstrual cycle:_____ Daytime activity:_____

Mid-day body temperature:_____ Time taken:_____

Mood Narrative:_____

_____

_____

_____

_____

Afternoon Energy level:_____Bowel movements:_____

_____

Headache/joint pain/other pain symptoms:_____

_____

_____

_____

_____

Exercise activity and duration:_____

Relaxation/restoration activities:_____

_____

Evening blue light blocking: Yes   No

Evening/Bedtime hunger:_____

Evening body temperature:_____   Time taken:_____

Bedtime:_____ Libido:_____

Nutrition:

Breakfast time:_____Food:_____

_____

Snack time:_____Food:_____

Lunch time:_____Food:_____

_____

Snack time:_____Food:_____

Dinner time:_____Food:_____

_____

Snack time:_____Food:_____

Daily water intake total:_____

Other notes:_____

_____

_____

_____

_____

_____

_____

_____

_____

Date:_____

Circadian Rhythm & Metabolic Clock:

Hours of sleep:_____Time it took to fall asleep:_____

Number of night wakings:_____

Explain any difficulty falling back asleep:_____

_____

Wake-up time:_____ Sleep quality:_____

_____

Wake up feeling rested: Yes   No

Morning body temperature: _____ Time taken: _____

Morning energy level:_____Morning sunlight:_____

Day of menstrual cycle:_____ Daytime activity:_____

Mid-day body temperature:_____ Time taken:_____

Mood Narrative:_____

_____

_____

_____

_____

Afternoon Energy level:_____Bowel movements:_____

_____

Headache/joint pain/other pain symptoms:_____

_____

_____

_____

_____

Exercise activity and duration:_____

Relaxation/restoration activities:_____

_____

Evening blue light blocking: Yes   No

Evening/Bedtime hunger:_____

Evening body temperature:_____   Time taken:_____

Bedtime:_____ Libido:_____

Nutrition:

Breakfast time:_____Food:_____

_____

Snack time:_____Food:_____

Lunch time:_____Food:_____

_____

Snack time:_____Food:_____

Dinner time:_____Food:_____

_____

Snack time:_____Food:_____

Daily water intake total:_____

Other notes:_____

_____

_____

_____

_____

_____

_____

_____

_____

Date:_____

Circadian Rhythm & Metabolic Clock:

Hours of sleep:_____Time it took to fall asleep:_____

Number of night wakings:_____

Explain any difficulty falling back asleep:_____

_____

Wake-up time:_____ Sleep quality:_____

_____

Wake up feeling rested: Yes   No

Morning body temperature: _____   Time taken: _____

Morning energy level:_____Morning sunlight:_____

Day of menstrual cycle:_____ Daytime activity:_____

Mid-day body temperature:_____ Time taken:_____

Mood Narrative:_____

_____

_____

_____

_____

Afternoon Energy level:_____Bowel movements:_____

_____

Headache/joint pain/other pain symptoms:_____

_____

_____

_____

_____

Exercise activity and duration:_____

Relaxation/restoration activities:_____

_____

Evening blue light blocking: Yes   No

Evening/Bedtime hunger:_____

Evening body temperature:_____   Time taken:_____

Bedtime:_____ Libido:_____

Nutrition:

Breakfast time:_____Food:_____

_____

Snack time:_____Food:_____

Lunch time:_____Food:_____

_____

Snack time:_____Food:_____

Dinner time:_____Food:_____

_____

Snack time:_____Food:_____

Daily water intake total:_____

Other notes:_____

_____

_____

_____

_____

_____

_____

_____

_____

Date:_____

Circadian Rhythm & Metabolic Clock:

Hours of sleep:_____Time it took to fall asleep:_____

Number of night wakings:_____

Explain any difficulty falling back asleep:_____

_____

Wake-up time:_____ Sleep quality:_____

_____

Wake up feeling rested: Yes   No

Morning body temperature: _____   Time taken: _____

Morning energy level:_____Morning sunlight:_____

Day of menstrual cycle:_____ Daytime activity:_____

Mid-day body temperature:_____ Time taken:_____

Mood Narrative:_____

_____

_____

_____

_____

Afternoon Energy level:_____Bowel movements:_____

_____

Headache/joint pain/other pain symptoms:_____

_____

_____

_____

_____

Exercise activity and duration:_____

30

Relaxation/restoration activities:_____

_____

Evening blue light blocking: Yes   No

Evening/Bedtime hunger:_____

Evening body temperature:_____   Time taken:_____

Bedtime:_____ Libido:_____

Nutrition:

Breakfast time:_____Food:_____

_____

Snack time:_____Food:_____

Lunch time:_____Food:_____

_____

Snack time:_____Food:_____

Dinner time:_____Food:_____

_____

Snack time:_____Food:_____

Daily water intake total:_____

Other notes:_____

_____

_____

_____

_____

_____

_____

_____

_____

Date:_____

Circadian Rhythm & Metabolic Clock:

Hours of sleep:_____Time it took to fall asleep:_____

Number of night wakings:_____

Explain any difficulty falling back asleep:_____

_____

Wake-up time:_____ Sleep quality:_____

_____

Wake up feeling rested: Yes   No

Morning body temperature: _____   Time taken: _____

Morning energy level:_____Morning sunlight:_____

Day of menstrual cycle:_____ Daytime activity:_____

Mid-day body temperature:_____ Time taken:_____

Mood Narrative:_____

_____

_____

_____

_____

Afternoon Energy level:_____Bowel movements:_____

_____

Headache/joint pain/other pain symptoms:_____

_____

_____

_____

_____

Exercise activity and duration:_____

Relaxation/restoration activities:_____

_____

Evening blue light blocking: Yes   No

Evening/Bedtime hunger:_____

Evening body temperature:_____   Time taken:_____

Bedtime:_____ Libido:_____

Nutrition:

Breakfast time:_____Food:_____

_____

Snack time:_____Food:_____

Lunch time:_____Food:_____

_____

Snack time:_____Food:_____

Dinner time:_____Food:_____

_____

Snack time:_____Food:_____

Daily water intake total:_____

Other notes:_____

_____

_____

_____

_____

_____

_____

_____

_____

Date:_____

Circadian Rhythm & Metabolic Clock:

Hours of sleep:_____Time it took to fall asleep:_____

Number of night wakings:_____

Explain any difficulty falling back asleep:_____

_____

Wake-up time:_____ Sleep quality:_____

_____

Wake up feeling rested: Yes   No

Morning body temperature: _____   Time taken: _____

Morning energy level:_____Morning sunlight:_____

Day of menstrual cycle:_____ Daytime activity:_____

Mid-day body temperature:_____ Time taken:_____

Mood Narrative:_____

_____

_____

_____

_____

Afternoon Energy level:_____Bowel movements:_____

_____

Headache/joint pain/other pain symptoms:_____

_____

_____

_____

_____

Exercise activity and duration:_____

Relaxation/restoration activities:_____

_____

Evening blue light blocking: Yes   No

Evening/Bedtime hunger:_____

Evening body temperature:_____   Time taken:_____

Bedtime:_____ Libido:_____

Nutrition:

Breakfast time:_____Food:_____

_____

Snack time:_____Food:_____

Lunch time:_____Food:_____

_____

Snack time:_____Food:_____

Dinner time:_____Food:_____

_____

Snack time:_____Food:_____

Daily water intake total:_____

Other notes:_____

_____

_____

_____

_____

_____

_____

_____

Week 2 Summary

What went well:_____
_____
_____
_____
_____
_____
_____

What didn't go so well:_____
_____
_____
_____
_____
_____

Any patterns or potential cause/effect relationships:_____
_____
_____
_____
_____

Questions to ask my doctor:_____
_____
_____

Week 3

Date:_____

Circadian Rhythm & Metabolic Clock:

Hours of sleep:_____Time it took to fall asleep:_____

Number of night wakings:_____

Explain any difficulty falling back asleep:_____

_____

Wake-up time:_____ Sleep quality:_____

_____

Wake up feeling rested: Yes   No

Morning body temperature: _____ Time taken: _____

Morning energy level:_____Morning sunlight:_____

Day of menstrual cycle:_____ Daytime activity:_____

Mid-day body temperature:_____ Time taken:_____

Mood Narrative:_____

_____

_____

_____

_____

Afternoon Energy level:_____Bowel movements:_____

_____

Headache/joint pain/other pain symptoms:_____

_____

_____

_____

_____

Exercise activity and duration:_____

Relaxation/restoration activities:_____

_____

Evening blue light blocking: Yes   No

Evening/Bedtime hunger:_____

Evening body temperature:_____   Time taken:_____

Bedtime:_____ Libido:_____

Nutrition:

Breakfast time:_____Food:_____

_____

Snack time:_____Food:_____

Lunch time:_____Food:_____

_____

Snack time:_____Food:_____

Dinner time:_____Food:_____

_____

Snack time:_____Food:_____

Daily water intake total:_____

Other notes:_____

_____

_____

_____

_____

_____

_____

_____

_____

Date:_____

Circadian Rhythm & Metabolic Clock:

Hours of sleep:_____Time it took to fall asleep:_____

Number of night wakings:_____

Explain any difficulty falling back asleep:_____

_____

Wake-up time:_____ Sleep quality:_____

_____

Wake up feeling rested: Yes   No

Morning body temperature: _____ Time taken: _____

Morning energy level:_____Morning sunlight:_____

Day of menstrual cycle:_____ Daytime activity:_____

Mid-day body temperature:_____ Time taken:_____

Mood Narrative:_____

_____

_____

_____

_____

Afternoon Energy level:_____Bowel movements:_____

_____

Headache/joint pain/other pain symptoms:_____

_____

_____

_____

_____

Exercise activity and duration:_____

Relaxation/restoration activities:_____

_____

Evening blue light blocking: Yes   No

Evening/Bedtime hunger:_____

Evening body temperature:_____ Time taken:_____

Bedtime:_____ Libido:_____

Nutrition:

Breakfast time:_____Food:_____

_____

Snack time:_____Food:_____

Lunch time:_____Food:_____

_____

Snack time:_____Food:_____

Dinner time:_____Food:_____

_____

Snack time:_____Food:_____

Daily water intake total:_____

Other notes:_____

_____

_____

_____

_____

_____

_____

_____

_____

Date:_____

Circadian Rhythm & Metabolic Clock:

Hours of sleep:_____Time it took to fall asleep:_____

Number of night wakings:_____

Explain any difficulty falling back asleep:_____

_____

Wake-up time:_____ Sleep quality:_____

_____

Wake up feeling rested: Yes   No

Morning body temperature: _____   Time taken: _____

Morning energy level:_____Morning sunlight:_____

Day of menstrual cycle:_____ Daytime activity:_____

Mid-day body temperature:_____ Time taken:_____

Mood Narrative:_____

_____

_____

_____

_____

Afternoon Energy level:_____Bowel movements:_____

_____

Headache/joint pain/other pain symptoms:_____

_____

_____

_____

_____

Exercise activity and duration:_____

Relaxation/restoration activities:_____

_____

Evening blue light blocking: Yes   No

Evening/Bedtime hunger:_____

Evening body temperature:_____   Time taken:_____

Bedtime:_____ Libido:_____

Nutrition:

Breakfast time:_____Food:_____

_____

Snack time:_____Food:_____

Lunch time:_____Food:_____

_____

Snack time:_____Food:_____

Dinner time:_____Food:_____

_____

Snack time:_____Food:_____

Daily water intake total:_____

Other notes:_____

_____

_____

_____

_____

_____

_____

_____

Date:_____

Circadian Rhythm & Metabolic Clock:

Hours of sleep:_____Time it took to fall asleep:_____

Number of night wakings:_____

Explain any difficulty falling back asleep:_____

_____

Wake-up time:_____ Sleep quality:_____

_____

Wake up feeling rested: Yes   No

Morning body temperature: _____   Time taken: _____

Morning energy level:_____Morning sunlight:_____

Day of menstrual cycle:_____ Daytime activity:_____

Mid-day body temperature:_____ Time taken:_____

Mood Narrative:_____

_____

_____

_____

_____

Afternoon Energy level:_____Bowel movements:_____

_____

Headache/joint pain/other pain symptoms:_____

_____

_____

_____

_____

Exercise activity and duration:_____

Relaxation/restoration activities:_____

_____

Evening blue light blocking: Yes   No

Evening/Bedtime hunger:_____

Evening body temperature:_____   Time taken:_____

Bedtime:_____ Libido:_____

Nutrition:

Breakfast time:_____Food:_____

_____

Snack time:_____Food:_____

Lunch time:_____Food:_____

_____

Snack time:_____Food:_____

Dinner time:_____Food:_____

_____

Snack time:_____Food:_____

Daily water intake total:_____

Other notes:_____

_____

_____

_____

_____

_____

_____

_____

_____

Date:_____

Circadian Rhythm & Metabolic Clock:

Hours of sleep:_____Time it took to fall asleep:_____

Number of night wakings:_____

Explain any difficulty falling back asleep:_____

_____

Wake-up time:_____ Sleep quality:_____

_____

Wake up feeling rested: Yes   No

Morning body temperature: _____   Time taken: _____

Morning energy level:_____Morning sunlight:_____

Day of menstrual cycle:_____ Daytime activity:_____

Mid-day body temperature:_____ Time taken:_____

Mood Narrative:_____

_____

_____

_____

_____

Afternoon Energy level:_____Bowel movements:_____

_____

Headache/joint pain/other pain symptoms:_____

_____

_____

_____

_____

Exercise activity and duration:_____

Relaxation/restoration activities:_____

_____

Evening blue light blocking: Yes   No

Evening/Bedtime hunger:_____

Evening body temperature:_____   Time taken:_____

Bedtime:_____ Libido:_____

Nutrition:

Breakfast time:_____Food:_____

_____

Snack time:_____Food:_____

Lunch time:_____Food:_____

_____

Snack time:_____Food:_____

Dinner time:_____Food:_____

_____

Snack time:_____Food:_____

Daily water intake total:_____

Other notes:_____

_____

_____

_____

_____

_____

_____

_____

Date:_____

Circadian Rhythm & Metabolic Clock:

Hours of sleep:_____Time it took to fall asleep:_____

Number of night wakings:_____

Explain any difficulty falling back asleep:_____

_____

Wake-up time:_____ Sleep quality:_____

_____

Wake up feeling rested: Yes   No

Morning body temperature: _____   Time taken: _____

Morning energy level:_____Morning sunlight:_____

Day of menstrual cycle:_____ Daytime activity:_____

Mid-day body temperature:_____ Time taken:_____

Mood Narrative:_____

_____

_____

_____

_____

Afternoon Energy level:_____Bowel movements:_____

_____

Headache/joint pain/other pain symptoms:_____

_____

_____

_____

_____

Exercise activity and duration:_____

Relaxation/restoration activities:_____

_____

Evening blue light blocking: Yes   No

Evening/Bedtime hunger:_____

Evening body temperature:_____   Time taken:_____

Bedtime:_____ Libido:_____

Nutrition:

Breakfast time:_____Food:_____

_____

Snack time:_____Food:_____

Lunch time:_____Food:_____

_____

Snack time:_____Food:_____

Dinner time:_____Food:_____

_____

Snack time:_____Food:_____

Daily water intake total:_____

Other notes:_____

_____

_____

_____

_____

_____

_____

_____

_____

Date:_____

Circadian Rhythm & Metabolic Clock:

Hours of sleep:_____Time it took to fall asleep:_____

Number of night wakings:_____

Explain any difficulty falling back asleep:_____

_____

Wake-up time:_____ Sleep quality:_____

_____

Wake up feeling rested: Yes   No

Morning body temperature: _____   Time taken: _____

Morning energy level:_____Morning sunlight:_____

Day of menstrual cycle:_____ Daytime activity:_____

Mid-day body temperature:_____ Time taken:_____

Mood Narrative:_____

_____

_____

_____

_____

Afternoon Energy level:_____Bowel movements:_____

_____

Headache/joint pain/other pain symptoms:_____

_____

_____

_____

_____

Exercise activity and duration:_____

Relaxation/restoration activities:_____

_____

Evening blue light blocking: Yes   No

Evening/Bedtime hunger:_____

Evening body temperature:_____   Time taken:_____

Bedtime:_____ Libido:_____

Nutrition:

Breakfast time:_____Food:_____

_____

Snack time:_____Food:_____

Lunch time:_____Food:_____

_____

Snack time:_____Food:_____

Dinner time:_____Food:_____

_____

Snack time:_____Food:_____

Daily water intake total:_____

Other notes:_____

_____

_____

_____

_____

_____

_____

_____

_____

Week 3 Summary

What went well:_____

_____

_____

_____

_____

_____

_____

What didn't go so well:_____

_____

_____

_____

_____

_____

Any patterns or potential cause/effect relationships:_____

_____

_____

_____

_____

Questions to ask my doctor:_____

_____

_____

Week 4

Date:_____

Body Composition & Measurements:
Chest:_____ Waist:_____

Bicep:_____ Hips:_____

Thigh:_____Calf:_____

Body Fat percentage:_____Weight:_____

Circadian Rhythm & Metabolic Clock

Hours of sleep:_____Time it took to fall asleep:_____

Number of night wakings:_____

Explain any difficulty falling back asleep:_____

_____

Wake-up time:_____ Sleep quality:_____

_____

Wake up feeling rested: Yes   No

Morning body temperature: _____   Time taken: _____

Morning energy level:_____Morning sunlight:_____

Day of menstrual cycle:_____ Daytime activity:_____

Mid-day body temperature:_____ Time taken:_____

Mood Narrative:_____

_____

_____

_____

Afternoon Energy level:_____Bowel movements:_____

_____

Headache/joint pain/other pain symptoms:_____

_____

_____

_____

_____

Exercise activity and duration:_____

Relaxation/restoration activities:_____

_____

Evening blue light blocking: Yes   No

Evening/Bedtime hunger:_____

Evening body temperature:_____   Time taken:_____

Bedtime:_____   Libido:_____

Nutrition:

Breakfast time:_____Food:_____

_____

Snack time:_____Food:_____

Lunch time:_____Food:_____

_____

Snack time:_____Food:_____

Dinner time:_____Food:_____

_____

Snack time:_____Food:_____

Daily water intake total:_____

Other notes:_____

_____

_____

_____

_____

Date:_____

Circadian Rhythm & Metabolic Clock:

Hours of sleep:_____Time it took to fall asleep:_____

Number of night wakings:_____

Explain any difficulty falling back asleep:_____

_____

Wake-up time:_____ Sleep quality:_____

_____

Wake up feeling rested: Yes   No

Morning body temperature: _____   Time taken: _____

Morning energy level:_____Morning sunlight:_____

Day of menstrual cycle:_____ Daytime activity:_____

Mid-day body temperature:_____   Time taken:_____

Mood Narrative:_____

_____

_____

_____

_____

Afternoon Energy level:_____Bowel movements:_____

_____

Headache/joint pain/other pain symptoms:_____

_____

_____

_____

_____

Exercise activity and duration:_____

Relaxation/restoration activities:_____

_____

Evening blue light blocking: Yes   No

Evening/Bedtime hunger:_____

Evening body temperature:_____   Time taken:_____

Bedtime:_____ Libido:_____

Nutrition:

Breakfast time:_____Food:_____

_____

Snack time:_____Food:_____

Lunch time:_____Food:_____

_____

Snack time:_____Food:_____

Dinner time:_____Food:_____

_____

Snack time:_____Food:_____

Daily water intake total:_____

Other notes:_____

_____

_____

_____

_____

_____

_____

_____

_____

Date:_____

Circadian Rhythm & Metabolic Clock:

Hours of sleep:_____Time it took to fall asleep:_____

Number of night wakings:_____

Explain any difficulty falling back asleep:_____

_____

Wake-up time:_____ Sleep quality:_____

_____

Wake up feeling rested: Yes   No

Morning body temperature: _____   Time taken: _____

Morning energy level:_____Morning sunlight:_____

Day of menstrual cycle:_____ Daytime activity:_____

Mid-day body temperature:_____ Time taken:_____

Mood Narrative:_____

_____

_____

_____

_____

Afternoon Energy level:_____Bowel movements:_____

_____

Headache/joint pain/other pain symptoms:_____

_____

_____

_____

_____

Exercise activity and duration:_____

Relaxation/restoration activities:_____

_____

Evening blue light blocking: Yes   No

Evening/Bedtime hunger:_____

Evening body temperature:_____   Time taken:_____

Bedtime:_____ Libido:_____

Nutrition:

Breakfast time:_____Food:_____

_____

Snack time:_____Food:_____

Lunch time:_____Food:_____

_____

Snack time:_____Food:_____

Dinner time:_____Food:_____

_____

Snack time:_____Food:_____

Daily water intake total:_____

Other notes:_____

_____

_____

_____

_____

_____

_____

_____

Date:_____

Circadian Rhythm & Metabolic Clock:

Hours of sleep:_____Time it took to fall asleep:_____

Number of night wakings:_____

Explain any difficulty falling back asleep:_____

_____

Wake-up time:_____ Sleep quality:_____

_____

Wake up feeling rested: Yes   No

Morning body temperature: _____   Time taken: _____

Morning energy level:_____Morning sunlight:_____

Day of menstrual cycle:_____ Daytime activity:_____

Mid-day body temperature:_____ Time taken:_____

Mood Narrative:_____

_____

_____

_____

_____

Afternoon Energy level:_____Bowel movements:_____

_____

Headache/joint pain/other pain symptoms:_____

_____

_____

_____

_____

Exercise activity and duration:_____

Relaxation/restoration activities:_____

_____

Evening blue light blocking: Yes   No

Evening/Bedtime hunger:_____

Evening body temperature:_____   Time taken:_____

Bedtime:_____ Libido:_____

Nutrition:

Breakfast time:_____Food:_____

_____

Snack time:_____Food:_____

Lunch time:_____Food:_____

_____

Snack time:_____Food:_____

Dinner time:_____Food:_____

_____

Snack time:_____Food:_____

Daily water intake total:_____

Other notes:_____

_____

_____

_____

_____

_____

_____

_____

Date:_____

Circadian Rhythm & Metabolic Clock:

Hours of sleep:_____Time it took to fall asleep:_____

Number of night wakings:_____

Explain any difficulty falling back asleep:_____

_____

Wake-up time:_____ Sleep quality:_____

_____

Wake up feeling rested: Yes   No

Morning body temperature: _____   Time taken: _____

Morning energy level:_____Morning sunlight:_____

Day of menstrual cycle:_____ Daytime activity:_____

Mid-day body temperature:_____ Time taken:_____

Mood Narrative:_____

_____

_____

_____

_____

Afternoon Energy level:_____Bowel movements:_____

_____

Headache/joint pain/other pain symptoms:_____

_____

_____

_____

_____

Exercise activity and duration:_____

Relaxation/restoration activities:_____

_____

Evening blue light blocking: Yes   No

Evening/Bedtime hunger:_____

Evening body temperature:_____   Time taken:_____

Bedtime:_____ Libido:_____

Nutrition:

Breakfast time:_____Food:_____

_____

Snack time:_____Food:_____

Lunch time:_____Food:_____

_____

Snack time:_____Food:_____

Dinner time:_____Food:_____

_____

Snack time:_____Food:_____

Daily water intake total:_____

Other notes:_____

_____

_____

_____

_____

_____

_____

_____

_____

Date:_____

Circadian Rhythm & Metabolic Clock:

Hours of sleep:_____Time it took to fall asleep:_____

Number of night wakings:_____

Explain any difficulty falling back asleep:_____

_____

Wake-up time:_____ Sleep quality:_____

_____

Wake up feeling rested: Yes   No

Morning body temperature: _____   Time taken: _____

Morning energy level:_____Morning sunlight:_____

Day of menstrual cycle:_____ Daytime activity:_____

Mid-day body temperature:_____ Time taken:_____

Mood Narrative:_____

_____

_____

_____

_____

Afternoon Energy level:_____Bowel movements:_____

_____

Headache/joint pain/other pain symptoms:_____

_____

_____

_____

_____

Exercise activity and duration:_____

Relaxation/restoration activities:_____

_____

Evening blue light blocking: Yes   No

Evening/Bedtime hunger:_____

Evening body temperature:_____   Time taken:_____

Bedtime:_____ Libido:_____

Nutrition:

Breakfast time:_____Food:_____

_____

Snack time:_____Food:_____

Lunch time:_____Food:_____

_____

Snack time:_____Food:_____

Dinner time:_____Food:_____

_____

Snack time:_____Food:_____

Daily water intake total:_____

Other notes:_____

_____

_____

_____

_____

_____

_____

_____

Date:_____

Circadian Rhythm & Metabolic Clock:

Hours of sleep:_____Time it took to fall asleep:_____

Number of night wakings:_____

Explain any difficulty falling back asleep:_____

_____

Wake-up time:_____ Sleep quality:_____

_____

Wake up feeling rested: Yes   No

Morning body temperature: _____   Time taken: _____

Morning energy level:_____Morning sunlight:_____

Day of menstrual cycle:_____ Daytime activity:_____

Mid-day body temperature:_____ Time taken:_____

Mood Narrative:_____

_____

_____

_____

_____

Afternoon Energy level:_____Bowel movements:_____

_____

Headache/joint pain/other pain symptoms:_____

_____

_____

_____

_____

Exercise activity and duration:_____

Relaxation/restoration activities:_____

_____

Evening blue light blocking: Yes   No

Evening/Bedtime hunger:_____

Evening body temperature:_____   Time taken:_____

Bedtime:_____ Libido:_____

Nutrition:

Breakfast time:_____Food:_____

_____

Snack time:_____Food:_____

Lunch time:_____Food:_____

_____

Snack time:_____Food:_____

Dinner time:_____Food:_____

_____

Snack time:_____Food:_____

Daily water intake total:_____

Other notes:_____

_____

_____

_____

_____

_____

_____

_____

_____

Week 4 Summary

What went well:_____

_____

_____

_____

_____

_____

What didn't go so well:_____

_____

_____

_____

_____

_____

Any patterns or potential cause/effect relationships:_____

_____

_____

_____

_____

_____

Questions to ask my doctor:_____

_____

_____

Week 5

Date:_____

Circadian Rhythm & Metabolic Clock:

Hours of sleep:_____Time it took to fall asleep:_____

Number of night wakings:_____

Explain any difficulty falling back asleep:_____

_____

Wake-up time:_____ Sleep quality:_____

_____

Wake up feeling rested: Yes   No

Morning body temperature: _____   Time taken: _____

Morning energy level:_____Morning sunlight:_____

Day of menstrual cycle:_____ Daytime activity:_____

Mid-day body temperature:_____ Time taken:_____

Mood Narrative:_____

_____

_____

_____

_____

Afternoon Energy level:_____Bowel movements:_____

_____

Headache/joint pain/other pain symptoms:_____

_____

_____

_____

_____

Exercise activity and duration:_____

Relaxation/restoration activities:_____

_____

Evening blue light blocking: Yes   No

Evening/Bedtime hunger:_____

Evening body temperature:_____   Time taken:_____

Bedtime:_____ Libido:_____

Nutrition:

Breakfast time:_____Food:_____

_____

Snack time:_____Food:_____

Lunch time:_____Food:_____

_____

Snack time:_____Food:_____

Dinner time:_____Food:_____

_____

Snack time:_____Food:_____

Daily water intake total:_____

Other notes:_____

_____

_____

_____

_____

_____

_____

_____

Date:_____

Circadian Rhythm & Metabolic Clock:

Hours of sleep:_____Time it took to fall asleep:_____

Number of night wakings:_____

Explain any difficulty falling back asleep:_____

_____

Wake-up time:_____ Sleep quality:_____

_____

Wake up feeling rested: Yes   No

Morning body temperature: _____   Time taken: _____

Morning energy level:_____Morning sunlight:_____

Day of menstrual cycle:_____ Daytime activity:_____

Mid-day body temperature:_____ Time taken:_____

Mood Narrative:_____

_____

_____

_____

Afternoon Energy level:_____Bowel movements:_____

_____

Headache/joint pain/other pain symptoms:_____

_____

_____

_____

_____

Exercise activity and duration:_____

Relaxation/restoration activities:_____

_____

Evening blue light blocking: Yes   No

Evening/Bedtime hunger:_____

Evening body temperature:_____   Time taken:_____

Bedtime:_____ Libido:_____

Nutrition:

Breakfast time:_____Food:_____

_____

Snack time:_____Food:_____

Lunch time:_____Food:_____

_____

Snack time:_____Food:_____

Dinner time:_____Food:_____

_____

Snack time:_____Food:_____

Daily water intake total:_____

Other notes:_____

_____

_____

_____

_____

_____

_____

_____

_____

Date:_____

Circadian Rhythm & Metabolic Clock:

Hours of sleep:_____Time it took to fall asleep:_____

Number of night wakings:_____

Explain any difficulty falling back asleep:_____

_____

Wake-up time:_____ Sleep quality:_____

_____

Wake up feeling rested: Yes   No

Morning body temperature: _____   Time taken: _____

Morning energy level:_____Morning sunlight:_____

Day of menstrual cycle:_____ Daytime activity:_____

Mid-day body temperature:_____ Time taken:_____

Mood Narrative:_____

_____

_____

_____

_____

Afternoon Energy level:_____Bowel movements:_____

_____

Headache/joint pain/other pain symptoms:_____

_____

_____

_____

_____

Exercise activity and duration:_____

Relaxation/restoration activities:_____

_____

Evening blue light blocking: Yes   No

Evening/Bedtime hunger:_____

Evening body temperature:_____   Time taken:_____

Bedtime:_____ Libido:_____

Nutrition:

Breakfast time:_____Food:_____

_____

Snack time:_____Food:_____

Lunch time:_____Food:_____

_____

Snack time:_____Food:_____

Dinner time:_____Food:_____

_____

Snack time:_____Food:_____

Daily water intake total:_____

Other notes:_____

_____

_____

_____

_____

_____

_____

_____

_____

Date:_____

Circadian Rhythm & Metabolic Clock:

Hours of sleep:_____Time it took to fall asleep:_____

Number of night wakings:_____

Explain any difficulty falling back asleep:_____

_____

Wake-up time:_____ Sleep quality:_____

_____

Wake up feeling rested: Yes   No

Morning body temperature: _____   Time taken: _____

Morning energy level:_____Morning sunlight:_____

Day of menstrual cycle:_____ Daytime activity:_____

Mid-day body temperature:_____ Time taken:_____

Mood Narrative:_____

_____

_____

_____

_____

Afternoon Energy level:_____Bowel movements:_____

_____

Headache/joint pain/other pain symptoms:_____

_____

_____

_____

_____

Exercise activity and duration:_____

Relaxation/restoration activities:_____

_____

Evening blue light blocking: Yes   No

Evening/Bedtime hunger:_____

Evening body temperature:_____   Time taken:_____

Bedtime:_____ Libido:_____

Nutrition:

Breakfast time:_____Food:_____

_____

Snack time:_____Food:_____

Lunch time:_____Food:_____

_____

Snack time:_____Food:_____

Dinner time:_____Food:_____

_____

Snack time:_____Food:_____

Daily water intake total:_____

Other notes:_____

_____

_____

_____

_____

_____

_____

_____

_____

Date:_____

Circadian Rhythm & Metabolic Clock:

Hours of sleep:_____Time it took to fall asleep:_____

Number of night wakings:_____

Explain any difficulty falling back asleep:_____

_____

Wake-up time:_____ Sleep quality:_____

_____

Wake up feeling rested: Yes   No

Morning body temperature: _____   Time taken: _____

Morning energy level:_____Morning sunlight:_____

Day of menstrual cycle:_____ Daytime activity:_____

Mid-day body temperature:_____ Time taken:_____

Mood Narrative:_____

_____

_____

_____

_____

Afternoon Energy level:_____Bowel movements:_____

_____

Headache/joint pain/other pain symptoms:_____

_____

_____

_____

_____

Exercise activity and duration:_____

Relaxation/restoration activities:_____

_____

Evening blue light blocking: Yes   No

Evening/Bedtime hunger:_____

Evening body temperature:_____   Time taken:_____

Bedtime:_____ Libido:_____

Nutrition:

Breakfast time:_____Food:_____

_____

Snack time:_____Food:_____

Lunch time:_____Food:_____

_____

Snack time:_____Food:_____

Dinner time:_____Food:_____

_____

Snack time:_____Food:_____

Daily water intake total:_____

Other notes:_____

_____

_____

_____

_____

_____

_____

_____

_____

Date:_____

Circadian Rhythm & Metabolic Clock:

Hours of sleep:_____Time it took to fall asleep:_____

Number of night wakings:_____

Explain any difficulty falling back asleep:_____

_____

Wake-up time:_____ Sleep quality:_____

_____

Wake up feeling rested: Yes   No

Morning body temperature: _____   Time taken: _____

Morning energy level:_____Morning sunlight:_____

Day of menstrual cycle:_____ Daytime activity:_____

Mid-day body temperature:_____ Time taken:_____

Mood Narrative:_____

_____

_____

_____

_____

Afternoon Energy level:_____Bowel movements:_____

_____

Headache/joint pain/other pain symptoms:_____

_____

_____

_____

_____

Exercise activity and duration:_____

Relaxation/restoration activities:_____

_____

Evening blue light blocking: Yes   No

Evening/Bedtime hunger:_____

Evening body temperature:_____   Time taken:_____

Bedtime:_____ Libido:_____

Nutrition:

Breakfast time:_____Food:_____

_____

Snack time:_____Food:_____

Lunch time:_____Food:_____

_____

Snack time:_____Food:_____

Dinner time:_____Food:_____

_____

Snack time:_____Food:_____

Daily water intake total:_____

Other notes:_____

_____

_____

_____

_____

_____

_____

_____

_____

Date:_____

Circadian Rhythm & Metabolic Clock:

Hours of sleep:_____Time it took to fall asleep:_____

Number of night wakings:_____

Explain any difficulty falling back asleep:_____

_____

Wake-up time:_____ Sleep quality:_____

_____

Wake up feeling rested: Yes   No

Morning body temperature: _____   Time taken: _____

Morning energy level:_____Morning sunlight:_____

Day of menstrual cycle:_____ Daytime activity:_____

Mid-day body temperature:_____ Time taken:_____

Mood Narrative:_____

_____

_____

_____

_____

Afternoon Energy level:_____Bowel movements:_____

_____

Headache/joint pain/other pain symptoms:_____

_____

_____

_____

_____

Exercise activity and duration:_____

Relaxation/restoration activities:_____

_____

Evening blue light blocking: Yes   No

Evening/Bedtime hunger:_____

Evening body temperature:_____   Time taken:_____

Bedtime:_____ Libido:_____

Nutrition:

Breakfast time:_____Food:_____

_____

Snack time:_____Food:_____

Lunch time:_____Food:_____

_____

Snack time:_____Food:_____

Dinner time:_____Food:_____

_____

Snack time:_____Food:_____

Daily water intake total:_____

Other notes:_____

_____

_____

_____

_____

_____

_____

_____

_____

Week 5 Summary

What went well:_____

_____

_____

_____

_____

_____

_____

What didn't go so well:_____

_____

_____

_____

_____

_____

Any patterns or potential cause/effect relationships:_____

_____

_____

_____

_____

Questions to ask my doctor:_____

_____

_____

Week 6

Date:_____

Circadian Rhythm & Metabolic Clock:

Hours of sleep:_____Time it took to fall asleep:_____

Number of night wakings:_____

Explain any difficulty falling back asleep:_____

_____

Wake-up time:_____ Sleep quality:_____

_____

Wake up feeling rested: Yes   No

Morning body temperature: _____   Time taken: _____

Morning energy level:_____Morning sunlight:_____

Day of menstrual cycle:_____ Daytime activity:_____

Mid-day body temperature:_____ Time taken:_____

Mood Narrative:_____

_____

_____

_____

_____

Afternoon Energy level:_____Bowel movements:_____

_____

Headache/joint pain/other pain symptoms:_____

_____

_____

_____

_____

Exercise activity and duration:_____

Relaxation/restoration activities:_____

_____

Evening blue light blocking: Yes   No

Evening/Bedtime hunger:_____

Evening body temperature:_____   Time taken:_____

Bedtime:_____ Libido:_____

Nutrition:

Breakfast time:_____Food:_____

_____

Snack time:_____Food:_____

Lunch time:_____Food:_____

_____

Snack time:_____Food:_____

Dinner time:_____Food:_____

_____

Snack time:_____Food:_____

Daily water intake total:_____

Other notes:_____

_____

_____

_____

_____

_____

_____

_____

Date:_____

Circadian Rhythm & Metabolic Clock:

Hours of sleep:_____Time it took to fall asleep:_____

Number of night wakings:_____

Explain any difficulty falling back asleep:_____

_____

Wake-up time:_____ Sleep quality:_____

_____

Wake up feeling rested: Yes   No

Morning body temperature: _____   Time taken: _____

Morning energy level:_____Morning sunlight:_____

Day of menstrual cycle:_____ Daytime activity:_____

Mid-day body temperature:_____ Time taken:_____

Mood Narrative:_____

_____

_____

_____

_____

Afternoon Energy level:_____Bowel movements:_____

_____

Headache/joint pain/other pain symptoms:_____

_____

_____

_____

_____

Exercise activity and duration:_____

Relaxation/restoration activities:_____

_____

Evening blue light blocking: Yes   No

Evening/Bedtime hunger:_____

Evening body temperature:_____   Time taken:_____

Bedtime:_____ Libido:_____

Nutrition:

Breakfast time:_____Food:_____

_____

Snack time:_____Food:_____

Lunch time:_____Food:_____

_____

Snack time:_____Food:_____

Dinner time:_____Food:_____

_____

Snack time:_____Food:_____

Daily water intake total:_____

Other notes:_____

_____

_____

_____

_____

_____

_____

_____

Date:_____

Circadian Rhythm & Metabolic Clock:

Hours of sleep:_____Time it took to fall asleep:_____

Number of night wakings:_____

Explain any difficulty falling back asleep:_____

_____

Wake-up time:_____ Sleep quality:_____

_____

Wake up feeling rested: Yes   No

Morning body temperature: _____   Time taken: _____

Morning energy level:_____Morning sunlight:_____

Day of menstrual cycle:_____ Daytime activity:_____

Mid-day body temperature:_____ Time taken:_____

Mood Narrative:_____

_____

_____

_____

_____

Afternoon Energy level:_____Bowel movements:_____

_____

Headache/joint pain/other pain symptoms:_____

_____

_____

_____

_____

Exercise activity and duration:_____

Relaxation/restoration activities:_____

_____

Evening blue light blocking: Yes   No

Evening/Bedtime hunger:_____

Evening body temperature:_____   Time taken:_____

Bedtime:_____ Libido:_____

Nutrition:

Breakfast time:_____Food:_____

_____

Snack time:_____Food:_____

Lunch time:_____Food:_____

_____

Snack time:_____Food:_____

Dinner time:_____Food:_____

_____

Snack time:_____Food:_____

Daily water intake total:_____

Other notes:_____

_____

_____

_____

_____

_____

_____

_____

Date:_____

Circadian Rhythm & Metabolic Clock:

Hours of sleep:_____Time it took to fall asleep:_____

Number of night wakings:_____

Explain any difficulty falling back asleep:_____

_____

Wake-up time:_____ Sleep quality:_____

_____

Wake up feeling rested: Yes   No

Morning body temperature: _____   Time taken: _____

Morning energy level:_____Morning sunlight:_____

Day of menstrual cycle:_____ Daytime activity:_____

Mid-day body temperature:_____ Time taken:_____

Mood Narrative:_____

_____

_____

_____

_____

Afternoon Energy level:_____Bowel movements:_____

_____

Headache/joint pain/other pain symptoms:_____

_____

_____

_____

_____

Exercise activity and duration:_____

Relaxation/restoration activities:_____

_____

Evening blue light blocking: Yes   No

Evening/Bedtime hunger:_____

Evening body temperature:_____   Time taken:_____

Bedtime:_____ Libido:_____

Nutrition:

Breakfast time:_____Food:_____

_____

Snack time:_____Food:_____

Lunch time:_____Food:_____

_____

Snack time:_____Food:_____

Dinner time:_____Food:_____

_____

Snack time:_____Food:_____

Daily water intake total:_____

Other notes:_____

_____

_____

_____

_____

_____

_____

_____

Date:_____

Circadian Rhythm & Metabolic Clock:

Hours of sleep:_____Time it took to fall asleep:_____

Number of night wakings:_____

Explain any difficulty falling back asleep:_____

_____

Wake-up time:_____ Sleep quality:_____

_____

Wake up feeling rested: Yes   No

Morning body temperature: _____   Time taken: _____

Morning energy level:_____Morning sunlight:_____

Day of menstrual cycle:_____ Daytime activity:_____

Mid-day body temperature:_____ Time taken:_____

Mood Narrative:_____

_____

_____

_____

_____

Afternoon Energy level:_____Bowel movements:_____

_____

Headache/joint pain/other pain symptoms:_____

_____

_____

_____

_____

Exercise activity and duration:_____

Relaxation/restoration activities:_____

_____

Evening blue light blocking: Yes   No

Evening/Bedtime hunger:_____

Evening body temperature:_____   Time taken:_____

Bedtime:_____ Libido:_____

Nutrition:

Breakfast time:_____Food:_____

_____

Snack time:_____Food:_____

Lunch time:_____Food:_____

_____

Snack time:_____Food:_____

Dinner time:_____Food:_____

_____

Snack time:_____Food:_____

Daily water intake total:_____

Other notes:_____

_____

_____

_____

_____

_____

_____

_____

_____

Date:_____

Circadian Rhythm & Metabolic Clock:

Hours of sleep:_____Time it took to fall asleep:_____

Number of night wakings:_____

Explain any difficulty falling back asleep:_____

_____

Wake-up time:_____ Sleep quality:_____

_____

Wake up feeling rested: Yes   No

Morning body temperature: _____   Time taken: _____

Morning energy level:_____Morning sunlight:_____

Day of menstrual cycle:_____ Daytime activity:_____

Mid-day body temperature:_____ Time taken:_____

Mood Narrative:_____

_____

_____

_____

_____

Afternoon Energy level:_____Bowel movements:_____

_____

Headache/joint pain/other pain symptoms:_____

_____

_____

_____

_____

Exercise activity and duration:_____

Relaxation/restoration activities:_____

_____

Evening blue light blocking: Yes   No

Evening/Bedtime hunger:_____

Evening body temperature:_____   Time taken:_____

Bedtime:_____ Libido:_____

Nutrition:

Breakfast time:_____Food:_____

_____

Snack time:_____Food:_____

Lunch time:_____Food:_____

_____

Snack time:_____Food:_____

Dinner time:_____Food:_____

_____

Snack time:_____Food:_____

Daily water intake total:_____

Other notes:_____

_____

_____

_____

_____

_____

_____

_____

_____

Date:_____

Circadian Rhythm & Metabolic Clock:

Hours of sleep:_____Time it took to fall asleep:_____

Number of night wakings:_____

Explain any difficulty falling back asleep:_____

_____

Wake-up time:_____ Sleep quality:_____

_____

Wake up feeling rested: Yes   No

Morning body temperature: _____   Time taken: _____

Morning energy level:_____Morning sunlight:_____

Day of menstrual cycle:_____ Daytime activity:_____

Mid-day body temperature:_____ Time taken:_____

Mood Narrative:_____

_____

_____

_____

_____

Afternoon Energy level:_____Bowel movements:_____

_____

Headache/joint pain/other pain symptoms:_____

_____

_____

_____

_____

Exercise activity and duration:_____

Relaxation/restoration activities:_____

_____

Evening blue light blocking: Yes   No

Evening/Bedtime hunger:_____

Evening body temperature:_____   Time taken:_____

Bedtime:_____ Libido:_____

Nutrition:

Breakfast time:_____Food:_____

_____

Snack time:_____Food:_____

Lunch time:_____Food:_____

_____

Snack time:_____Food:_____

Dinner time:_____Food:_____

_____

Snack time:_____Food:_____

Daily water intake total:_____

Other notes:_____

_____

_____

_____

_____

_____

_____

_____

_____

Week 6 Summary

What went well:_____

_____

_____

_____

_____

_____

_____

What didn't go so well:_____

_____

_____

_____

_____

_____

_____

Any patterns or potential cause/effect relationships:_____

_____

_____

_____

_____

_____

Questions to ask my doctor:_____

_____

_____

Week 7

Date:_____

Circadian Rhythm & Metabolic Clock:

Hours of sleep:_____Time it took to fall asleep:_____

Number of night wakings:_____

Explain any difficulty falling back asleep:_____

_____

Wake-up time:_____ Sleep quality:_____

_____

Wake up feeling rested: Yes   No

Morning body temperature: _____   Time taken: _____

Morning energy level:_____Morning sunlight:_____

Day of menstrual cycle:_____ Daytime activity:_____

Mid-day body temperature:_____ Time taken:_____

Mood Narrative:_____

_____

_____

_____

_____

Afternoon Energy level:_____Bowel movements:_____

_____

Headache/joint pain/other pain symptoms:_____

_____

_____

_____

_____

Exercise activity and duration:_____

Relaxation/restoration activities:_____

_____

Evening blue light blocking: Yes   No

Evening/Bedtime hunger:_____

Evening body temperature:_____   Time taken:_____

Bedtime:_____ Libido:_____

Nutrition:

Breakfast time:_____Food:_____

_____

Snack time:_____Food:_____

Lunch time:_____Food:_____

_____

Snack time:_____Food:_____

Dinner time:_____Food:_____

_____

Snack time:_____Food:_____

Daily water intake total:_____

Other notes:_____

_____

_____

_____

_____

_____

_____

_____

_____

Date:_____

Circadian Rhythm & Metabolic Clock:

Hours of sleep:_____Time it took to fall asleep:_____

Number of night wakings:_____

Explain any difficulty falling back asleep:_____

_____

Wake-up time:_____ Sleep quality:_____

_____

Wake up feeling rested: Yes   No

Morning body temperature: _____   Time taken: _____

Morning energy level:_____Morning sunlight:_____

Day of menstrual cycle:_____ Daytime activity:_____

Mid-day body temperature:_____ Time taken:_____

Mood Narrative:_____

_____

_____

_____

_____

Afternoon Energy level:_____Bowel movements:_____

_____

Headache/joint pain/other pain symptoms:_____

_____

_____

_____

_____

Exercise activity and duration:_____

Relaxation/restoration activities:_____

_____

Evening blue light blocking: Yes   No

Evening/Bedtime hunger:_____

Evening body temperature:_____   Time taken:_____

Bedtime:_____   Libido:_____

Nutrition:

Breakfast time:_____Food:_____

_____

Snack time:_____Food:_____

Lunch time:_____Food:_____

_____

Snack time:_____Food:_____

Dinner time:_____Food:_____

_____

Snack time:_____Food:_____

Daily water intake total:_____

Other notes:_____

_____

_____

_____

_____

_____

_____

_____

Date:_____

Circadian Rhythm & Metabolic Clock:

Hours of sleep:_____Time it took to fall asleep:_____

Number of night wakings:_____

Explain any difficulty falling back asleep:_____

_____

Wake-up time:_____ Sleep quality:_____

_____

Wake up feeling rested: Yes   No

Morning body temperature: _____   Time taken: _____

Morning energy level:_____Morning sunlight:_____

Day of menstrual cycle:_____ Daytime activity:_____

Mid-day body temperature:_____ Time taken:_____

Mood Narrative:_____

_____

_____

_____

Afternoon Energy level:_____Bowel movements:_____

_____

Headache/joint pain/other pain symptoms:_____

_____

_____

_____

_____

Exercise activity and duration:_____

Relaxation/restoration activities:_____

_____

Evening blue light blocking: Yes   No

Evening/Bedtime hunger:_____

Evening body temperature:_____   Time taken:_____

Bedtime:_____ Libido:_____

Nutrition:

Breakfast time:_____Food:_____

_____

Snack time:_____Food:_____

Lunch time:_____Food:_____

_____

Snack time:_____Food:_____

Dinner time:_____Food:_____

_____

Snack time:_____Food:_____

Daily water intake total:_____

Other notes:_____

_____

_____

_____

_____

_____

_____

_____

Date:_____

Circadian Rhythm & Metabolic Clock:

Hours of sleep:_____Time it took to fall asleep:_____

Number of night wakings:_____

Explain any difficulty falling back asleep:_____

_____

Wake-up time:_____ Sleep quality:_____

_____

Wake up feeling rested: Yes   No

Morning body temperature: _____   Time taken: _____

Morning energy level:_____Morning sunlight:_____

Day of menstrual cycle:_____ Daytime activity:_____

Mid-day body temperature:_____ Time taken:_____

Mood Narrative:_____

_____

_____

_____

_____

Afternoon Energy level:_____Bowel movements:_____

_____

Headache/joint pain/other pain symptoms:_____

_____

_____

_____

_____

Exercise activity and duration:_____

Relaxation/restoration activities:_____

_____

Evening blue light blocking: Yes   No

Evening/Bedtime hunger:_____

Evening body temperature:_____   Time taken:_____

Bedtime:_____ Libido:_____

Nutrition:

Breakfast time:_____Food:_____

_____

Snack time:_____Food:_____

Lunch time:_____Food:_____

_____

Snack time:_____Food:_____

Dinner time:_____Food:_____

_____

Snack time:_____Food:_____

Daily water intake total:_____

Other notes:_____

_____

_____

_____

_____

_____

_____

_____

_____

Date:_____

Circadian Rhythm & Metabolic Clock:

Hours of sleep:_____Time it took to fall asleep:_____

Number of night wakings:_____

Explain any difficulty falling back asleep:_____

_____

Wake-up time:_____ Sleep quality:_____

_____

Wake up feeling rested: Yes   No

Morning body temperature: _____   Time taken: _____

Morning energy level:_____Morning sunlight:_____

Day of menstrual cycle:_____ Daytime activity:_____

Mid-day body temperature:_____ Time taken:_____

Mood Narrative:_____

_____

_____

_____

_____

Afternoon Energy level:_____Bowel movements:_____

_____

Headache/joint pain/other pain symptoms:_____

_____

_____

_____

_____

Exercise activity and duration:_____

Relaxation/restoration activities:_____

_____

Evening blue light blocking: Yes   No

Evening/Bedtime hunger:_____

Evening body temperature:_____   Time taken:_____

Bedtime:_____ Libido:_____

Nutrition:

Breakfast time:_____Food:_____

_____

Snack time:_____Food:_____

Lunch time:_____Food:_____

_____

Snack time:_____Food:_____

Dinner time:_____Food:_____

_____

Snack time:_____Food:_____

Daily water intake total:_____

Other notes:_____

_____

_____

_____

_____

_____

_____

_____

Date:_____

Circadian Rhythm & Metabolic Clock:

Hours of sleep:_____ Time it took to fall asleep:_____

Number of night wakings:_____

Explain any difficulty falling back asleep:_____

_____

Wake-up time:_____ Sleep quality:_____

_____

Wake up feeling rested: Yes   No

Morning body temperature: _____   Time taken: _____

Morning energy level:_____Morning sunlight:_____

Day of menstrual cycle:_____ Daytime activity:_____

Mid-day body temperature:_____ Time taken:_____

Mood Narrative:_____

_____

_____

_____

_____

Afternoon Energy level:_____Bowel movements:_____

_____

Headache/joint pain/other pain symptoms:_____

_____

_____

_____

_____

Exercise activity and duration:_____

Relaxation/restoration activities:_____

_____

Evening blue light blocking: Yes   No

Evening/Bedtime hunger:_____

Evening body temperature:_____   Time taken:_____

Bedtime:_____ Libido:_____

Nutrition:

Breakfast time:_____Food:_____

_____

Snack time:_____Food:_____

Lunch time:_____Food:_____

_____

Snack time:_____Food:_____

Dinner time:_____Food:_____

_____

Snack time:_____Food:_____

Daily water intake total:_____

Other notes:_____

_____

_____

_____

_____

_____

_____

_____

_____

Date:_____

Circadian Rhythm & Metabolic Clock:

Hours of sleep:_____Time it took to fall asleep:_____

Number of night wakings:_____

Explain any difficulty falling back asleep:_____

_____

Wake-up time:_____ Sleep quality:_____

_____

Wake up feeling rested: Yes   No

Morning body temperature: _____   Time taken: _____

Morning energy level:_____Morning sunlight:_____

Day of menstrual cycle:_____ Daytime activity:_____

Mid-day body temperature:_____ Time taken:_____

Mood Narrative:_____

_____

_____

_____

_____

Afternoon Energy level:_____Bowel movements:_____

_____

Headache/joint pain/other pain symptoms:_____

_____

_____

_____

_____

Exercise activity and duration:_____

Relaxation/restoration activities:_____
_____

Evening blue light blocking: Yes   No

Evening/Bedtime hunger:_____

Evening body temperature:_____   Time taken:_____

Bedtime:_____ Libido:_____

Nutrition:

Breakfast time:_____Food:_____
_____

Snack time:_____Food:_____

Lunch time:_____Food:_____
_____

Snack time:_____Food:_____

Dinner time:_____Food:_____
_____

Snack time:_____Food:_____

Daily water intake total:_____

Other notes:_____
_____
_____
_____
_____
_____
_____
_____
_____

Week 7 Summary

What went well:_____
_____
_____
_____
_____
_____
_____

What didn't go so well:_____
_____
_____
_____
_____
_____

Any patterns or potential cause/effect relationships:_____
_____
_____
_____
_____
_____

Questions to ask my doctor:_____
_____
_____

Week 8

Date:_____

Body Composition & Measurements:
Chest:_____ Waist:_____

Bicep:_____ Hips:_____

Thigh:_____Calf:_____

Body Fat percentage:_____Weight:_____

Circadian Rhythm & Metabolic Clock:

Hours of sleep:_____Time it took to fall asleep:_____

Number of night wakings:_____

Explain any difficulty falling back asleep:_____

_____

Wake-up time:_____ Sleep quality:_____

_____

Wake up feeling rested: Yes   No

Morning body temperature: _____   Time taken: _____

Morning energy level:_____Morning sunlight:_____

Day of menstrual cycle:_____ Daytime activity:_____

Mid-day body temperature:_____ Time taken:_____

Mood Narrative:_____

_____

_____

_____

Afternoon Energy level:_____Bowel movements:_____

_____

Headache/joint pain/other pain symptoms:_____

_____

_____

_____

_____

Exercise activity and duration:_____

Relaxation/restoration activities:_____

_____

Evening blue light blocking: Yes   No

Evening/Bedtime hunger:_____

Evening body temperature:_____   Time taken:_____

Bedtime:_____ Libido:_____

Nutrition:

Breakfast time:_____Food:_____

_____

Snack time:_____Food:_____

Lunch time:_____Food:_____

_____

Snack time:_____Food:_____

Dinner time:_____Food:_____

_____

Snack time:_____Food:_____

Daily water intake total:_____

Other notes:_____

_____

_____

_____

_____

Date:_____

Circadian Rhythm & Metabolic Clock:

Hours of sleep:_____Time it took to fall asleep:_____

Number of night wakings:_____

Explain any difficulty falling back asleep:_____

_____

Wake-up time:_____ Sleep quality:_____

_____

Wake up feeling rested: Yes   No

Morning body temperature: _____   Time taken: _____

Morning energy level:_____Morning sunlight:_____

Day of menstrual cycle:_____ Daytime activity:_____

Mid-day body temperature:_____ Time taken:_____

Mood Narrative:_____

_____

_____

_____

_____

Afternoon Energy level:_____Bowel movements:_____

_____

Headache/joint pain/other pain symptoms:_____

_____

_____

_____

_____

Exercise activity and duration:_____

Relaxation/restoration activities:_____

_____

Evening blue light blocking: Yes   No

Evening/Bedtime hunger:_____

Evening body temperature:_____   Time taken:_____

Bedtime:_____ Libido:_____

Nutrition:

Breakfast time:_____Food:_____

_____

Snack time:_____Food:_____

Lunch time:_____Food:_____

_____

Snack time:_____Food:_____

Dinner time:_____Food:_____

_____

Snack time:_____Food:_____

Daily water intake total:_____

Other notes:_____

_____

_____

_____

_____

_____

_____

_____

Date:_____

Circadian Rhythm & Metabolic Clock:

Hours of sleep:_____Time it took to fall asleep:_____

Number of night wakings:_____

Explain any difficulty falling back asleep:_____

_____

Wake-up time:_____ Sleep quality:_____

_____

Wake up feeling rested: Yes   No

Morning body temperature: _____   Time taken: _____

Morning energy level:_____Morning sunlight:_____

Day of menstrual cycle:_____ Daytime activity:_____

Mid-day body temperature:_____ Time taken:_____

Mood Narrative:_____

_____

_____

_____

_____

Afternoon Energy level:_____Bowel movements:_____

_____

Headache/joint pain/other pain symptoms:_____

_____

_____

_____

_____

Exercise activity and duration:_____

Relaxation/restoration activities:_____

_____

Evening blue light blocking: Yes   No

Evening/Bedtime hunger:_____

Evening body temperature:_____   Time taken:_____

Bedtime:_____ Libido:_____

Nutrition:

Breakfast time:_____Food:_____

_____

Snack time:_____Food:_____

Lunch time:_____Food:_____

_____

Snack time:_____Food:_____

Dinner time:_____Food:_____

_____

Snack time:_____Food:_____

Daily water intake total:_____

Other notes:_____

_____

_____

_____

_____

_____

_____

_____

Date:_____

Circadian Rhythm & Metabolic Clock:

Hours of sleep:_____Time it took to fall asleep:_____

Number of night wakings:_____

Explain any difficulty falling back asleep:_____

_____

Wake-up time:_____ Sleep quality:_____

_____

Wake up feeling rested: Yes   No

Morning body temperature: _____   Time taken: _____

Morning energy level:_____Morning sunlight:_____

Day of menstrual cycle:_____ Daytime activity:_____

Mid-day body temperature:_____ Time taken:_____

Mood Narrative:_____

_____

_____

_____

_____

Afternoon Energy level:_____Bowel movements:_____

_____

Headache/joint pain/other pain symptoms:_____

_____

_____

_____

_____

Exercise activity and duration:_____

Relaxation/restoration activities:_____

_____

Evening blue light blocking: Yes   No

Evening/Bedtime hunger:_____

Evening body temperature:_____   Time taken:_____

Bedtime:_____ Libido:_____

Nutrition:

Breakfast time:_____Food:_____

_____

Snack time:_____Food:_____

Lunch time:_____Food:_____

_____

Snack time:_____Food:_____

Dinner time:_____Food:_____

_____

Snack time:_____Food:_____

Daily water intake total:_____

Other notes:_____

_____

_____

_____

_____

_____

_____

_____

Date:_____

Circadian Rhythm & Metabolic Clock:

Hours of sleep:_____Time it took to fall asleep:_____

Number of night wakings:_____

Explain any difficulty falling back asleep:_____

_____

Wake-up time:_____ Sleep quality:_____

_____

Wake up feeling rested: Yes   No

Morning body temperature: _____   Time taken: _____

Morning energy level:_____Morning sunlight:_____

Day of menstrual cycle:_____ Daytime activity:_____

Mid-day body temperature:_____ Time taken:_____

Mood Narrative:_____

_____

_____

_____

_____

Afternoon Energy level:_____Bowel movements:_____

_____

Headache/joint pain/other pain symptoms:_____

_____

_____

_____

_____

Exercise activity and duration:_____

Relaxation/restoration activities:_____

_____

Evening blue light blocking: Yes   No

Evening/Bedtime hunger:_____

Evening body temperature:_____   Time taken:_____

Bedtime:_____ Libido:_____

Nutrition:

Breakfast time:_____Food:_____

_____

Snack time:_____Food:_____

Lunch time:_____Food:_____

_____

Snack time:_____Food:_____

Dinner time:_____Food:_____

_____

Snack time:_____Food:_____

Daily water intake total:_____

Other notes:_____

_____

_____

_____

_____

_____

_____

_____

Date:_____

Circadian Rhythm & Metabolic Clock:

Hours of sleep:_____Time it took to fall asleep:_____

Number of night wakings:_____

Explain any difficulty falling back asleep:_____

_____

Wake-up time:_____ Sleep quality:_____

_____

Wake up feeling rested: Yes   No

Morning body temperature: _____   Time taken: _____

Morning energy level:_____Morning sunlight:_____

Day of menstrual cycle:_____ Daytime activity:_____

Mid-day body temperature:_____ Time taken:_____

Mood Narrative:_____

_____

_____

_____

_____

Afternoon Energy level:_____Bowel movements:_____

_____

Headache/joint pain/other pain symptoms:_____

_____

_____

_____

_____

Exercise activity and duration:_____

Relaxation/restoration activities:_____

_____

Evening blue light blocking: Yes   No

Evening/Bedtime hunger:_____

Evening body temperature:_____   Time taken:_____

Bedtime:_____ Libido:_____

Nutrition:

Breakfast time:_____Food:_____

_____

Snack time:_____Food:_____

Lunch time:_____Food:_____

_____

Snack time:_____Food:_____

Dinner time:_____Food:_____

_____

Snack time:_____Food:_____

Daily water intake total:_____

Other notes:_____

_____

_____

_____

_____

_____

_____

_____

Date:_____

Body Composition & Measurements:

Chest:_____ Waist:_____

Bicep:_____ Hips:_____

Thigh:_____ Calf:_____

Body Fat percentage:_____Weight:_____

Circadian Rhythm & Metabolic Clock:

Hours of sleep:_____Time it took to fall asleep:_____

Number of night wakings:_____

Explain any difficulty falling back asleep:_____

_____

Wake-up time:_____ Sleep quality:_____

_____

Wake up feeling rested: Yes   No

Morning body temperature: _____   Time taken: _____

Morning energy level:_____Morning sunlight:_____

Day of menstrual cycle:_____ Daytime activity:_____

Mid-day body temperature:_____ Time taken:_____

Mood Narrative:_____

_____

_____

_____

Afternoon Energy level:_____Bowel movements:_____

_____

Headache/joint pain/other pain symptoms:_____

_____

_____

_____

_____

Exercise activity and duration:_____

Relaxation/restoration activities:_____

_____

Evening blue light blocking: Yes   No

Evening/Bedtime hunger:_____

Evening body temperature:_____   Time taken:_____

Bedtime:_____ Libido:_____

Nutrition:

Breakfast time:_____Food:_____

_____

Snack time:_____Food:_____

Lunch time:_____Food:_____

_____

Snack time:_____Food:_____

Dinner time:_____Food:_____

_____

Snack time:_____Food:_____

Daily water intake total:_____

Other notes:_____

_____

_____

_____

_____

Week 8 Summary

What went well:_____

_____

_____

_____

_____

_____

_____

What didn't go so well:_____

_____

_____

_____

_____

_____

_____

Any patterns or potential cause/effect relationships:_____

_____

_____

_____

_____

_____

Questions to ask my doctor:_____

_____

_____

Use this space to reflect on any trends or other discoveries you have made over the past eight weeks:

_____

_____

_____

_____

_____

_____

_____

_____

_____

_____

_____

_____

_____

_____

_____

_____

_____

_____

_____

_____

_____

_____

_____

_____

_____

_____

_____

About the Author

Rachel Russell makes her home in the Pacific Northwest where she enjoys researching, writing, time with her family, and horseback riding. She is passionate about wellness and holistic health.

Connect with her at: www.soulsparkpublication.com for tips, tricks, and freebies.

Like this journal? Please leave a review on Amazon.com and share your experience with others.

This title is also available in spiral-bound form at TheBookPatch.com.